CONTENTS

REIKI FOR BEGINNERS

The comprehensive Beginner's Guide to Learn Reiki,
Self Healing and improve your energy level.

by Healeanor Crystal

Introduction

Reiki is a Japanese healing technique that is used to aid the body's natural healing ability, stress reduction and relaxation. It is administered by "laying on hands" to transmit the unseen "life force energy" that flows through us and into a patient. If a person's "life force energy" is low, then they are more likely to get sick or feel stress. Where as if it is high, they are more likely to be happy and healthy. Reiki is an intelligent energy that knows to target the area where healing needs to happen. Reiki knows to bring harmony back where harmony is lost. It is important to know as a practitioner not to force a Reiki treatment. Reiki will bring the results that are needed, not what you try to force.

For this reason it is important to remember that as a practitioner, it is your job to transmit this life force into a recipients bodies, even concentrating on specific areas. However it is not your job to control what Reiki does. Reiki will flow in accordance to the highest benefit of the recipient. Reiki will flow and heal with the ultimate purpose of restoring harmony.

It is also important to remember that a practitioner should be trying to heal the source of the problem, not the symptoms. This should be the intention and front of mind whenever a Reiki healing session is taking place. For example, imagine a person with back pain seeks out a Reiki healing session. Is it more prudent to just concentrate on pain relief, or to heal the source of this pain? Remember that removing the cause also removes the effect.

Symptoms may not disappear straight away, it's important that a person receiving Reiki understands this. Do not be discouraged and keep attending Reiki sessions. Time is a healer and it's important to remember this when having Reiki administered. Reiki for beginners primarily focusses on self-healing. As you progress through your Reiki journey you may want to learn about administering Reiki to someone else. This happens after Reiki level 2 where you will become attuned to performing Reiki on other people. It is important to remember that when you offer Reiki to someone else that you correctly explain the nature of Reiki healing.

This is basically explaining what you learnt above. Reiki heals sources, not symptoms. This will not happen right away but may take many Reiki sessions to fully address the root of the problem.

Secondly it is important to make a patient fully aware of the 'cleansing period'. This is very similar to what you yourself experienced after attunement in Reiki for beginners level 1, or even after level 2. Symptoms can grow stronger as the patient's body and mind joins in with the self-healing mechanics of Reiki. Explain that a person can experience changes across their life and that sometimes these may be intensive. They may notice signs in their lives that tell them what paths or directions they should be taking, what is not aiding their lives in anyway and would be better off stopped, who contributes and who takes away from their lives. It is important to explain these in detail otherwise a patient might get scared and stop Reiki treatment.

Also, try to determine if a person really wishes to be healed. Some people just don't want to get better for whatever reason. Have a long discussion with the patient and determine what their intentions are. If a person does not wish to be healed then Reiki will not have an effect on them. Whether you are interested in finding a practitioner to receive Reiki treatment, or you're seeking a practitioner to receive training, it's important to have a general idea what to expect. First, recognize that Reiki is not a cure-all answer to health and wellness. It is commonly referred to as "laying of hands," a process by which practitioner channels the natural life force energy that surrounds us, into a subject (I say subject because it works on all living things, not just humans).

This treatment is offered as a compliment to several methods of healing. It works on both the physical and metaphysical body to remove blockages of energy within the system.

To receive treatment requires the permission of the subject. Even when we do not realize it, if we are uncertain of our surroundings, we create blockages which prevent energy from reaching us. A subject must be willing to accept the energy in order for it to work. Most practitioners also require payment for their service.

This is commonly made in the form of money, but special arrangements are sometimes made for a different exchange. The point of this "exchange" is to serve as a balance for the energy transferred.

We tend to think of "energy" as a free-flowing, usually invisible field around us. Yet the purpose of Reiki is to provide balance to that field. This requires an exchange be made as "payment" for receipt of this energy. It is no different than receiving a gift for one's birthday, and sending a card to say "thank you" in acknowledgement of the gift. How you and your practitioner define "payment" is at your discretion.

Training in Reiki is a different path. It is becoming easier to search online and find classes offered by Reiki Masters where one may become certified in Reiki. Again, these classes are often compensated for with payment in the form of money. However, the payment for the class is up to an agreement between the Master and the student.

Usually there is more than one student in a class. This is very beneficial because each practitioner experiences this journey in his or her own way. It is important for each student to witness the experience of others to gain understanding of this journey. In turn, they will be able to relate to their subjects as they are treated, and experience different results

Some trainings usually take a whole year while you meet once in a month for several hours at a time. This, just as any other practice, is not something learned over night. It requires study, patience and ultimately a willingness to use what's been learned for the betterment of those around you. If you are considering taking a class to become a practitioner, I encourage you to speak with the teacher for some time before choosing to commit to the process. Reiki healing is very easy. Reiki Healing and Love will flow without any effort on your part. Place your hands on you self and others and experience Reiki Healing for yourself. How you begin your practice of Reiki is up to you as there are no set in rules for learning Reiki.

During the Reiki Attunement or after being attuned in Reiki you may notice "Sensations of energy, light, colors, or just feelings of general positivity and peace, or you may experience particularly vivid dreams. However it is perfectly ok to have noticed nothing unusual yet, as these sensations are not an indication that the attunements have been given. We always experience the Reiki Energy in our own unique way, and you may only start to experience it consciously after some practice."

History and Origin of Reiki

The Reiki method of healing was founded on the revelation and understanding of the body's energy system. Reiki Practitioners strive to improve health and *q*uality of life by offering Reiki energy and restoring balance. Reiki is used in self-care, for care of one's family, and is offered in private practice and in hospitals and medical settings as an adjunct and supportive therapy to wellness and traditional medical care. The form of Reiki that many people practice today, Usui Reiki, has been in use for over one hundred years.

The Founder of Reiki

The history of Usui Reiki begins with its founder, Dr. Mikao Usui. Sometimes called the Usui Sensei, Dr. Mikao Usui was born to a wealthy Buddhist family in 1865. Dr. Usui's family was able to give their son a well-rounded education for the time. As a child, Dr. Usui studied in a Buddhist monastery where he was taught martial arts, swordsmanship, and the Japanese form of Chi Kung, known as Kiko.

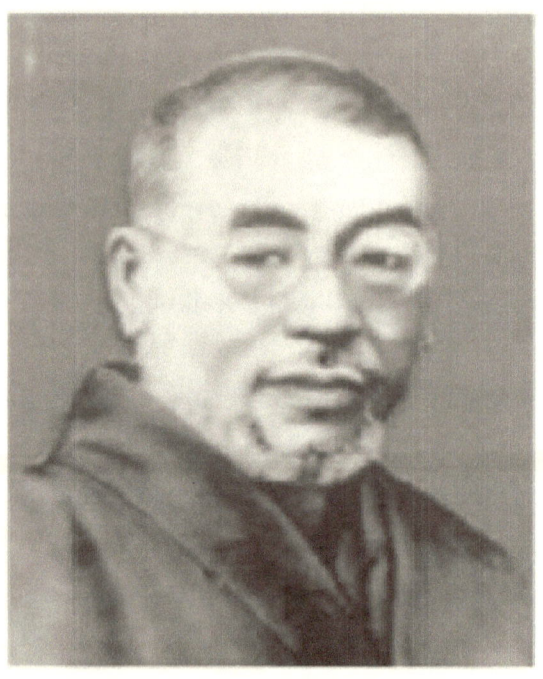

Throughout his education, Dr. Usui had an interest in medicine, psychology and theology. It was this interest that prompted him to seek a way to heal himself and others using the laying on of hands. It was his desire to find a method of healing that was unattached to any specific religion and religious belief, so that his system would be accessible to everyone.

Dr. Usui traveled a great deal during his lifetime. He studied healing systems of all types and held different professions including reporter, secretary, missionary, public servant and guard. Finally, he became a Buddhist priest/monk and lived in a monastery.

The Spiritual Awakening and Development of Reiki

Sometime during his years of training in the monastery, Dr. Usui attended his own training rediscovery course in a cave on Mount Kurama. For 21 days, Dr. Usui fasted, meditated and prayed. On

the morning of the twenty-first day, Dr. Usui experienced an event that would change his life forever. He saw ancient Sanskrit symbols that helped him develop the system of healing he had been struggling to invent. Usui Reiki was born.

After his spiritual awakening on Mount Kurama, Dr. Usui established a clinic for healing and teaching in Kyoto. As the practice of Usui Reiki was spreading, Dr. Usui became known for his healing practice.

Further development of Reiki

Mikao Usui founded his first Reiki clinic and school in Tokyo in 1922. Before he died, Dr. Usui taught several Reiki masters to ensure that his system would not be forgotten. Among them was Dr. Chujiro Hayashi, a former naval officer who set up a Reiki clinic in Tokyo.

Dr. Hayashi is credited with further developing the Usui system of Reiki by adding hand positions to more thoroughly cover the body. Dr. Hayashi also changed and refined the attunement process. Using his improved system, Dr. Hayashi trained several more Reiki Masters, including a woman named Hawayo Takata. Mrs. Takata was a Japanese-American woman who originally went to Dr. Hayashi for healing. Upon learning the system herself, Mrs. Takata took Reiki home to the United States.

Spread of Reiki to the West: Hawayo Takata was Tokyo in 1935. Mrs. Takata was very ill and in need of surgery, but she strongly felt through her instinct that she didn't need that surgery to be healed. After asking her doctor about alternative treatments for her condition, she was told about the Reiki practitioner in town. Mrs. Takata had never heard of Reiki, but she made an appointment, even though she was slightly skeptical. Following her initial meeting with Dr. Hayashi, Mrs. Takata saw Dr. Hayashi on a daily basis. She found the sessions to be relaxing and pleasant and, ultimately, healing.

As time passed, Mrs. Takata learned Reiki One and Reiki Two. When she returned to the United States, Mrs. Takata continued to practice Reiki and eventually became a Reiki Master. Much of this happened near the beginning of World War II.

Mrs. Takata wanted to spread her system of healing to others. She made changes to her Reiki practice, then used Reiki to help heal others in the United States.

Modern Reiki

Before he died, Dr. Hayashi managed to impart all of Dr. Usui's teachings onto Mrs. Takata. She continued to practice Reiki for many years. When she died, she had attuned 22 Reiki masters.

Today, people who practice Reiki use the methods developed by Dr. Usui, the founder of Usui Reiki. The genius of Reiki is that practitioners can utilize Reiki to help heal themselves and for their own wellness and enhanced well-being. In fact, working on self-healing is a prerequisite for offering Reiki healing to others. Modern Reiki masters can offer the Reiki energy to others through gentle static light pressure touch using the specific traditional Reiki hand positions and even over long distances like prayer is offered. Reiki healing complements many medicinal therapies and traditional medicine and can be used to help assist in the potential healing of people suffering from pain, illness, disease and more. Modern Reiki is becoming more popular as time goes on, and the lineage of Reiki masters is growing every day. With the return to Usui Reiki, many people are using this traditional hands on therapy to heal themselves and others

The Basics of Reiki

Reiki is an energy healing art which is so ancient that we don't actually know when or how it began. What is known is that has been around for thousands of years, apparently first developed in Tibet, and it was practiced by the shaman of each area or tribe, and was handed down from generation to generation. Sadly, this powerful healing art remained known in only that small portion of the earth, and was not even widely known in Tibet in recent centuries. In the 1800's, a man in Japan named Dr. Mikao Usui devoted nearly 30 years of his life, studying with the Reiki masters in Tibet, as well as studying other energy healing arts in various places, including pranic energy healing in India. He revived Reiki as a healing art, and he became widely known in Japan for his powerful healing treatments which were as effective as acupuncture. He began training other people in the art of Reiki healing, and opened a clinic which became extraordinarily successful. Dr. Usui's form of Reiki is known as Usui Reiki (no surprise!), and it is now the most common form, although Tibetan Reiki is increasingly more common. The first Westerner that studied at Dr.

Usui's clinic was a lady from the U.S. (Hawaii) named Hawayo Takata, who studied Reiki in Japan in the 1930's, but who only began to teach it to others much later in the 1970's (in Hawaii). From there, it spread to the mainland U.S. and beyond to the world. Since the 1970's, Reiki has become ever more widely accepted as a legitimate and effective method of healing by the traditional world of medicine. Reiki is offered these days in major hospitals around the U.S. and other countries, including prestigious Harvard University Medical School Hospital.

How does Reiki work?

Reiki treatments, as practiced in major hospitals, clinics, and by individual Reiki Masters, are effectively applied in order to:

❖   Treat the symptoms and the causes of illness

❖   Promote natural self-healing of injuries

❖   Strengthen the immune system

❖   Balance the energies of your body's organs and functions, to promote wellness

❖   Release blocked or suppressed feelings, to promote emotional & spiritual peace

❖   Enhance your ability to meditate

❖   Enhance spiritual growth and self-awareness and creativity

❖   Balance your energy centers (chakras, aura) for general Well-Being, happiness, empowerment

❖   Relaxes you and reduce stress

❖   Help you love yourself more

❖   Help you love your inner child more

❖   Balance & strengthen your emotional state

❖   Promote self-power through the power of love

❖   Promotes self confidence

"Rei" means Universe, or God Consciousness. "Ki" means Chi, or Life Force Energy.

"Reiki" means, basically, the life force energy of the universe, or of God (in Japanese).The Life Force Energy of the Universe is all around us, in us, moving through us, it is us, it is God, it is the Source of everything that exists, it is our very reason for existing, it is the very energy that is life.

Quantum physics (since Einstein 100 years ago) says that everything, is ONLY pure energy, and that what we see as the physical world is ONLY an illusion. That the physical world, our body, are things that we actually create to appear the way that they do, at every moment that we look at things or ourselves.

Quantum physics has proven that we ourselves are ONLY pure energy, that the physical being that we see in the mirror is only an illusion, that we are ONLY energy. It has proven that we are composed of the same exact energy that makes up the entire universe, which is the energy of the Source of life itself. Reiki treatments focus this universal life force energy (Chi) on your body and your spiritual being, allowing you to receive additional life force energy.

This strengthens the body and your emotional state in order to promote self-healing, it reduces stress, brings emotional balance and deep peaceful relaxation. Reiki enables a better quality of life as a result. Reiki is similar to other ancient energy healing arts such as traditional   Chinese acupuncture, Chi Gong, Tai Chi, Hindu Pranic Healing, and others. It is also known to be a way of gaining powerful spiritual development as well as impressive personal growth.

A Reiki Master treats the fully-clothed patient by placing his hands in 12 positions along the energy pathways and energy centers of your body which correspond to your energy system. These energy centers are called Chakras. The hand positions that are similar to some of the places of focus in acupuncture.

For a Reiki Distance healing, I place my hands in these positions on you in a virtual way, while you're on the phone with me, or while you're meditating, or even while you're sleeping. A Reiki Master does not use their human energy for healing - we channel directly from the benevolent nourishing Universal Source, the Life Force Energy of the Universe, of God.In addition to the powerful Reiki Healing techniques and symbols, use your psychic skills of vividly tapping into Source, and shamanic breathing (holotropic breathing), to strengthen the amount and the intensity of the nurturing blissfully euphoric healing energy that I channel into your being.

How to increase your power

Be in a quiet, meditative place without interruptions. Let go of any thoughts, and allow yourself to just FEEL good – feel the blissful connection to Source, to God, to Goddess, that you likely remember having felt before, feel it now. Visualize the space around you filled with sparkling, euphoric, blissful, love-filled, light, the energy of The Creator, the energy of Source. Know that you are also made up of this same energy, just as everything in the entire universe is pure energy in its essence.

Be aware of the 3 feet of space in all directions around you, which is the boundary of your own energy space, the edge of the energy that is you - a large cocoon-shaped space of energy, 3 feet in all directions.

Own it powerfully, be it intensely, and fill that space up with as much awareness and strength and power and intensity and density of being YOU that you can imagine!! Focus for at least 60 seconds on making the energy space that is you, as densely filled with your being and your energy, as you can imagine – make the light be as thick as gel.

Then, be aware of the room that you are in, and expand into the room, and fill ALL of the room with the same level of awareness and strength and power and intensity and density of being YOU that you can imagine!! Feel what it's like to touch that cold hard corner of the ceiling, BE the whole room, fill it with YOU as thick as gel. NOW, bring ALL of that energy which just filled the room, back into just the 3-feet cocoon-like energy space that is YOU. Notice how much stronger you feel, that you're lighter, more confident, more connected to Source. Next, expand into TWO rooms, fill them BOTH with that same level of awareness and strength and power and intensity and density of being YOU that you can imagine.

Feel what it's like to touch that piece of furniture in the next room, or the lamp fixture on the ceiling of this room, BE the whole of both rooms, fill them with YOU as thick as gel. NOW, bring ALL of THAT energy back into just the 3-feet cocoon-like energy space that is YOU. Notice how you feel even more powerful, more strong, even more light, more confident, more connected to Source!!You can keep expanding to your whole apartment (or house), then back to your 3-foot space, then your whole block, and back to your 3-foot space, then your whole neighbo-rhood, and back to your 3-foot space, etc. You can keep this up until you're filling the planet, the solar system, the galaxy, etc.

You will find this very effective and powerful.

How to Love and connect with your Inner Child

Sometimes we are aware if the feelings that weren't loved enough when we were very young in those years when our personality was being formed and solidified. This exercise allows you to go back in time and bring that missing love to your 5-year old self. This works because, in truth, time does not exist, we can change the past, change our perceptions. Be in a quiet, meditative place without interruptions.

Let go of any thoughts, and allow yourself to just FEEL good – feel the blissful connection to Source, to God, to Goddess, that you likely remember having felt before, feel it now. Sit in a chair, hold a pillow in your lap. Then, visualize, and FEEL, the pillow as 5-yr old YOU, on your lap, hold her in your arms, put your cheek gently down on the top of his head, say to her "I love you", say it with passion, FEEL how precious and innocent and sweet you were at that age, feel yourself as that beautiful little one, say to yourself "you are so beautiful, baby, you are precious, so pure, so sweet, so gentle, wanting so much just to be loved. Say to yourself, with so much passion, feeling, power and depth as you can allow yourself to feel.

Benefits and Limits of Reiki

Reiki is said to have multiple benefits and is applied for different needs, especially for clearing and tuning the chakras. One person may have a Reiki session to find relaxation from stress. A cancer patient might receive Reiki as a way to receive healing from the source. Some believe this energy comes from a higher power while others feel it comes from within. Despite these differences, many have experienced healing and the positive effects of Reiki.

Relieves pain, anxiety and fatigue

According to a review of randomized trials, reiki may help to reduce pain and anxiety, though more research is needed. It may also help to reduce fatigue.A 2015 study found that people being treated for cancer who received distant reiki in addition to regular medical care had lower levels of pain, anxiety, and fatigue. The use of reiki had been compared to physiotherapy for relieving lower back pain in people with herniated disk, both treatments were found to be equally effective at relieving back pains but reiki was more cost-effective and in some cases resulted in faster treatment.

Treats depression

Reiki treatments may be used as part of a treatment plan to help relieve depression. Researchers looked at the effects of reiki on older adults experiencing pain, depression, or anxiety and it reported an improvement on ones symptoms, mood and well-being. Reiki also brings about more feelings of relaxation, increased curiousity and enhances level of self-care.

Enhances quality of life

The positive benefits of reiki can enhance your overall well-being. Researchers has found out that reiki was helpful in improving the quality of life for women with cancer. Women who had reiki showed improvements to their sleep patterns, self-confidence, and depression levels. They noted a sense of calm, inner peace, and relaxation.

Boost moods

Reiki may help to improve your mood by relieving anxiety and depression. People who had reiki felt greater mood benefits compared to people who didn't have reiki. Reiki participants in a study who had six 30-minute sessions over a period of two to eight weeks showed improvements in their mood.

May improve some symptoms and conditions: Reiki may also be used to treat

- ❖ Headache

- ❖ Tension

- ❖ Insomnia

- ❖ Nausea

The relaxation response that happens with Reiki may benefit these symptoms. However, specific research is needed to determine the efficacy of reiki for the treatment of these symptoms and conditions.

May improve Memory and Behaviour

Reiki sessions has helped to improve the Behaviour and memory of people as a study that involves 24 patients with mild cognitive impairment and or and mild alzheimer's disease were carried out and reiki helped to improve their behavior greatly.

Reiki speeds up recovery from surgery or long-term illness

As it helps in adjusting to medicine/treatment, it also tends to reduce side-effects. For example, Chemo-therapy patients who received Reiki noticed a marked decrease in side effects from treatment.

Reiki can be an effective way to treat immediate problems

such as physical or mental illness (recovery from surgery, but regular treatments can also improve overall health. By helping to maintain a state of physical and emotional balance, Reiki can not only treat problems, but perhaps even prevent them from ever developing.

Limitations of Reiki

Just like the benefits of reiki there are also limitations, the limitations sometimes isn't through the lack of power but by the lack of imagination on the parts of some practitioners. Imagination is both creative and experimental; a part of the mind that we use used to develop theories and ideas which are vital to our development in the way we accomplish what we already know whilst developing new ways of doing things. The limits of reiki are stated below;

❖ Recipients absence or lack of receptiveness

❖ Channel could be limited to begin with, although channels get stronger with time and practice

❖ Regular sessions are desirable

❖ Cannot give distance treatment

❖ Needs other treatment in addition to reiki incase of serious illness

❖ Deliberate refusal of healing

❖ Should not be applied as sole treatment in acute emergencies but it's an excellent support in emergency nterventions

❖ Will need other form of treatments in addition to reiki in cases of serious illness

❖ Incase regular sessions are not possible the effect may not be very prominent

Reiki symbols and their unique uses

Many Reiki Masters consider the Reiki symbols holy and persist in the old Reiki tradition that they must be kept secret. The symbols should only be available to those who have been initiated at the Reiki 2 level. Many people today feel that this approach is no longer relevant as the symbols have been described in many books and freely available on the Internet. However, it is also believed the Reiki symbols and the information that can be read about them are of little value on their own.

In different tests it has been proven that the symbols have little or no use before a Reiki initiation. Students with no Reiki experience (but with psychic abilities) have been asked to memorize the symbols and then use them. The results differ from a control group will had the Reiki 2 initiation. The conclusion has been that it is the Reiki initiation as suchthat gives the Reiki symbols their power.The Reiki symbols are like keys which open doors to a higher mind. You can also see them as buttons, when you press the button, you automatically get a result. The symbols trigger a belief or intention built into the symbols to help the user to get the results intended. The different symbols also quickly connect the user to the universal life force. When a Reiki Master does an attunement and shows the symbols to the student, the form of the symbol is impressed in the mind and merges with the metaphysical energies it represents. When a Reiki practitioner draws, thinks about or visualizes a symbol, it instantly connects to the energies it represents.

Today, there are many different forms of Reiki, and some have incorporated their own symbols in the initiations. In "traditional" Reiki, there are three Reiki symbols given during the Reiki attunement. They are: The Power Symbol (Choku Rei) The Mental/Emotional Symbol (Sei He Ki) The Distance Symbol (Hon Sha Ze Sho Nen). The Reiki symbols are partly based on the Japanese writing system, Kanji. The symbols should be drawn or visualized as they have been taught during a Reiki 2 attunement. As more and more people get attuned to Reiki, this means that there can be a great number of variations between symbols taught by different Masters. This is not really a problem as there is not 100% right or wrong way to draw them. The Reiki symbols given to a student will work however they look, as they incorporate the intention and the connection to the metaphysical energies they represent. Having said that, it is our belief that it is essential to keep as much as is physically possible to the original symbols as distortions over time are symptomatic of our need for healing in the first place.

THE REIKI POWER SYMBOL

OF CHOKU REI

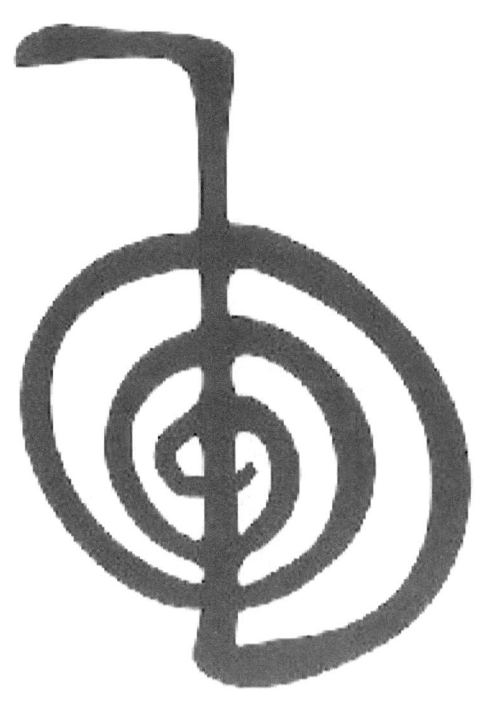

The general meaning of Choku Rei (pronounced Cho-Koo-Ray) is "place the power of the universe here". The Power Symbol can be used to increase the power of Reiki, or it can be used for protection. See it as a light switch that has the intention to instantly boost your ability to channel Reiki. Draw or visualize the symbol in front of you and you will have instant access to more healing energies. Choku Rei also gives the other symbols more power when they are used together. The symbol can be used at any time during a treatment, but it is especially effective if it is used at the beginning of a session or when used at the end of a session to close and seal off the Reiki energies.

Remember it is always your intention that governs what happens. If you want to add new functions to the Power Symbol, then just have a clear statement and intention of what you want the symbol to do and it will do it for you.

USES OF CHOKU REI

- Increase the power of your healing abilities; use it as a light switch. (Draw or visualize Choku Rei in front of you or draw it in your hands if you want). * You can focus the Reiki energies (like a looking glass) on a specific point of the body. (Draw the symbol directly on the spot being treated).
- Increase the power of the other symbols. (Draw it before drawing the other symbols). * One can use the Power Symbol to close the space around the recipient. (Draw it above the body with the intention of sealing the process).
- The Power Symbol can be used to spiritually clean a room from negative energies. (Draw or visualize the Symbol on all the walls, ceiling and floor with the intention to protect and energize the room).
- You can clean crystals and other objects from negative energies. (Draw the Power Symbol above or on the Crystal/object with the intention of cleansing it and restoring it to its original state. Hold the object in your hands and give it Reiki (or send it Reiki from a distance if the object is far away or too big to hold).

- Protect yourself from negative energies (from people you treat or from people you meet). Draw or visualize the Reiki Power Symbol in front of you with the intention of being totally protected.
- Protect yourself, your children, your spouse, your house and other things you value. (Draw Choku Rei directly on the objects/person you want to protect with the intention to protect him/her from harm. Since Reiki works on all different levels of existence, it will naturally also given protection on all levels of existence.

There are no limits to what you can do. The power is all in your mind - let your clear intention guide the function of the symbols.

THE REIKI MENTAL/EMO-
TIONAL SYMBOLS- SEI HE KI

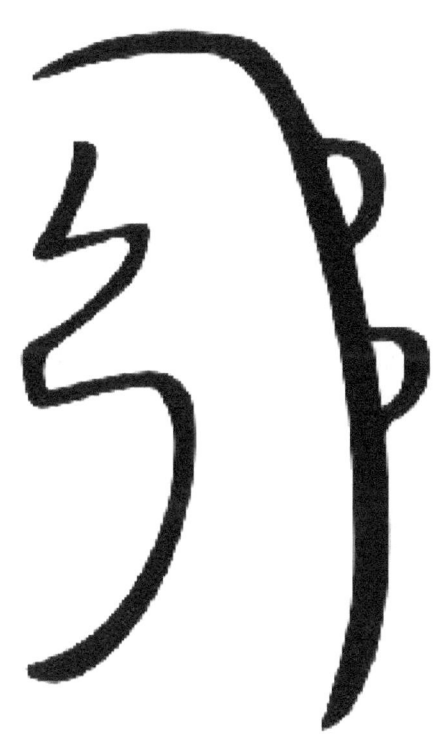

Sei He Ki (pronounced Say-Hay-Key) has a general meaning of "God and Man become one". The Mental/Emotional symbol brings together the "brain and the body". It helps people to bring to the surface and release the mental/emotional causes of their problems. Many people (even doctors) are starting to realize that many of our ailments are based on mental and emotional imbalances.

The symbol works to focus and harmonize the subconscious with the physical side. It can be used to help with emotional and mental healing. It balances the left and right side of the brain and gives peace and harmony. It is also very effective at relationship problems. The symbol can also be used on diverse problems like nervousness, fear, depression, anger, sadness etc.

USES OF SEE HE KI

- The symbols can be used to help overcome misuse of drugs, alcohol, smoking, etc.
- Sei He Ki can be used to lose weight.
- The symbol can be used to find things that you have misplaced. (Draw the symbol in front of you and ask for help in finding the object. Let go of trying, the answer will soon pop up).
- Sei He Ki can be used to improve your memory when reading or studying. (Draw the symbol on each page as you read it with the intention of remembering the important parts).
- Add the symbol with doing healing (normal or distance) as this can help the healing process. Many physical problems have mental/emotional roots.

The Mental/Emotional Symbol, Sei He Ki, has to do with Yin and Yang and the balance between the two sides of the brain. The left part of the symbol represents Yang and our left side of the brain (logic, structure and linear thinking etc).

The right side of this symbol represents Yin and our right side of the brain (fantasy, feelings, intuition, etc).

THE REIKI DISTANCE HEA-
LING SYMBOL - HON SHA ZE
SHO NEN

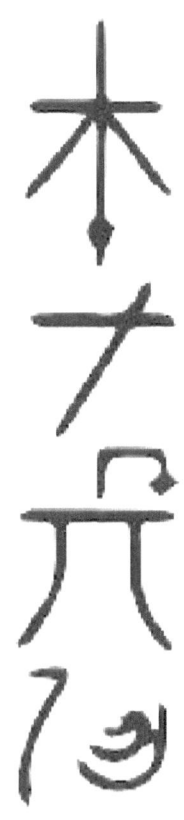

Hon Sha Ze Sho Nen (pronounced Hon-Sha-Zee-Show-Nen) has the general meaning of "No Past, No Present, No Future" or it could have the meaning of "The Buddha in me contacts the Buddha in you". This symbol can, as its name implies, be used to send energies over a distance.

Many practitioners consider Hon sha Ze Sho Nen as the most useful and powerful symbol. The use of this symbol gives access to the Akashic Records, the life records of each soul and can therefore be used in Karmic Healing. Trauma and other experiences from this life, previous or parallel lives that affect and mirror peoples' behaviors can be brought to light and released with this symbol.

In doing distance healing – be open! Do not focus your efforts on healing a specific problem like a headache. Send the Reiki energies without limitation, as they will go where they are best needed. When doing distance healing the energies will work at the receiver's subtle body, the chakras and the aura, and not as much of the physical level (i.e. It can take some time before the energies seep down to the body and ease the pain). The person you are sending Reiki to, is likely to feel it happening. If he/she has an open mind, he/she can usually tell what you have done and when you have done it.

Distance healing does not take nearly as long as a hands-on treatment. Only a few minutes are needed to send distance healing. You can even set up a Reiki distance healing to automatically repeat sending energies to a person. If you want to do this, we recommend that you put a time limit on the repeat (as it otherwise might continue forever), and also to review and empower the distance healing every other day. Remember, it is your intention that guides what happens.

- Send Reiki healing to people far away.
- "Beam" Reiki to people across the room.
- Send Reiki energies to the future to help with a specific task, or be there as a support.
- Send Reiki to the past to lift up, to understand and release trauma.

Absentee healing is basically a process of visualization, imagine or "see" the person you want to send healing to and just do it. You can use a photo if you have one, if not don't worry about it, just send it. Sometimes, we send to people we don't really know (like a name we have received in an e-mail request), we only have their name and city. No problem - it is the intention of sending Reiki to this unknown person that makes it work. Our advice is to let go of all your doubts. Use the Reiki symbols and send the energies.

How Reiki Healing works with the 5 Elements

Reiki practitioners use their hands to deliver energy and improve the flow and balance of the recipient's energy to support healing. Reiki assists in balancing your physical, mental, emotional and spiritual well-being to promote a deep sense of relaxation.

You may experience the energy as sensations such as heat, tingling, or pulsing where the practitioner places her hands on your body, or you may feel these sensations move through your body to other locations. Some people may not perceive any change at all.

Most people feel very relaxed and peaceful; many clients even fall asleep while receiving a Reiki treatment. During a Reiki session, you usually lie on a massage table or sit in a chair, fully clothed.

The Reiki practitioner uses light touch or non-touch and gently places his or her hands on or hovering above your body in specific energy locations during the session. The length of time that the practitioner leaves his or her hands in each position is determined by the flow of energy through his or her hands to you at each location.

There is no pressure, massage or manipulation.

Reiki heals by flowing through the affected parts of the energy field and charging them with positive energy. It raises the vibratory level of the energy field in and around the physical body where the negative thoughts and feelings are attached. This causes the negative energy to break apart and fall away. In so doing, Reiki clears, straightens and heals the energy pathways, thus allowing the life force to flow in a healthy and natural way. Reiki healing works with a system of energy healing that allows the practitioner to access the energies of the five elements to bring about healing and balance for oneself and for others. It works well by itself.

The spiritual healing art of Reiki works by channeling positive energy into your body, with Reiki masters and practitioners typically placing their hands on the affected areas of the body that need a boost, offering this energy and your body takes in the energy where most needed. This powerful flow of positive energy may bring a near immediate sensation of relief as it releases tension, lessens the impact of stress and replaces negative energy with the positive. Some refer to this positive Reiki energy as the life force, and indeed it can bring new life to a stressed-out, tired body.

The concept of the five elements of reiki in healing is elusive to some. To the hardened rational mind, it may seem to be an imaginary "placebo" concept for something that does not exist; or something that science has "just not explained" yet. To put it simply, the five elements of reiki in healing is a life force. It is the motivating energy, or force that is between pure, non-material thought, and manifest matter. The elements are the carrier wave of our spiritual intention.

Everything that happens in our universe involves the movement of these elements in some way. As we become more lovingly connected to our spirit and energy, and the spirit and energy that nourishes all life, our spiritual intention becomes more and more focused, and we are less concerned with our little "self". We feel and experience a greater connection to the events in our lives because our awareness is also increasing. When all this happens, our chi becomes more powerful, and this power is beyond anything physical. For many, this experience is the beginning of true healing.

In a practical sense, reiki healing assumes whatever qualities that are needed in order to carry out a particular task, purpose, or embodiment. Put another way, reiki healing in a real sense, becomes self-identical to that which it manifests as, and carries the potential to become. One of the primary formations of reiki healing that we know of is the Five Elements.

The five elements

Using each of these five elements individually is a strong practice yet when you combine them they produce a complete spiritual teaching that is accessible to everyone.

Each element supports the other, filling in the gaps that will exist for different practitioners. No two people have the same needs when learning. For this reason working with all five elements gives each practitioner a greater chance of success. Together these elements create a whole that is firm yet flexible, supporting practitioners on their individual spiritual paths.

The five elements are Wood, Fire, Earth, Metal, and Water. The element names are not meant to be taken literally, but their qualities are indeed reflected in the literal elements they are named after.

At the level of physical embodiment, each element is simply a particular way in which our life energy, or chi, manifests itself in order to accomplish a particu-

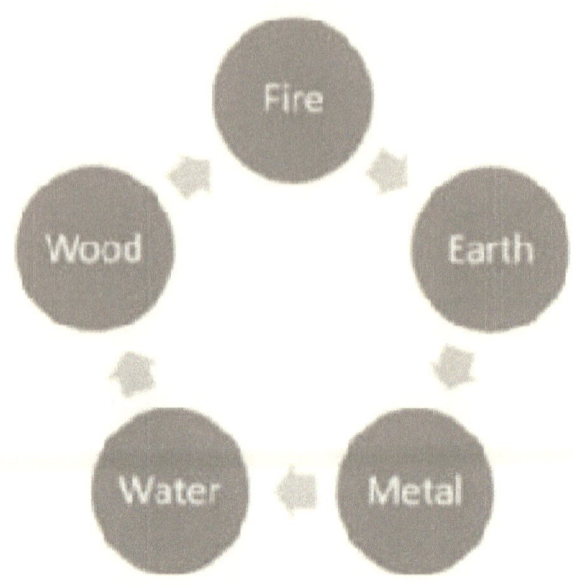

lar task that is necessary to our existence. It is only when we can no longer take in, or "ingest" these energies of life that we begin to have problems. Wherever an inability to take in our life force occurs in any one element, our emotional maturity, mental discernment, physical health, happiness and spiritual life will eventually suffer if we do not correct it.

This is because each element supports all the others and the whole by doing what it is supposed to do.

Think of the five elements as interdependent energies, all moving in a cycle that keeps transforming our overall life force in an alchemical fusion of creative expansion with Yang energy, and formative contraction with Yin energy. In other words, each element transforms into the next one after it through what it produces as it moves through our energy system. This transformation is all about bringing potential into manifestation in stages according to intent.

The fundamental way of explaining this is: Water (most Yin) creates Wood (Yang emerging) by nourishing it.

Wood feeds Fire (most Yang) by being fuel, Fire produces Earth (Yin/Yang balance) as ash (through combustion).

Earth produces Metal (Yin emerging) as minerals (ore), and Metal feeds Water (most Yin) by becoming condensed essential fluid (earth's core is molten iron, mercury is liquid at lower temperatures, for example).

Then, the process repeats with a new set of conditions. The expansion of our creative life force takes our overall life theme through a process of creative expression in the expansion phase, then culls the aspects that we let go of, and keeps the essence that is left from a given cycle in the contraction phase.

It all starts over again, but from the new time perspective of our life's unfoldment, and what we have "learned" from experience.

This unfolding is continuous in small and large increments of "time", and we experience it as our life spontaneously happening, day to day, week to week, month to month, and year to year.

This rhythm through time is why we see repeating patterns of events and behavior in our lives, and is key to resolving unwanted patterns in all areas of our existence at the human level.

In other words, our unconscious life patterns are rooted in our "undigested" elemental energies.

When examined closely, it will be seen that the metaphor is very accurate. It describes phenomena, which exists, and can be predicted in every strata of nature. Five Element theory energetically describes the function of our organs, and even the seasons of the Earth.

Five Element theory can be, and is, used in medical diagnosis. Although, it can be applied to psychology, spirituality, and even science; as well as healing work of all kinds. It is not the province of any single discipline.

INDIVIDUAL ELEMENTS

- **Water:** The Water element is reflected in the energy of winter. It is the essence of your will power, and the potential of manifestation in your life. Your ability to draw vitality from your life essence is a primary focus of the water element. The Water element meridians are the Bladder and Kidney meridians. Water is gentle when in balance, and fearful when not in balance.

- **Wood:** The Wood element is reflected in the energy of spring, and empowers your vision and perspective to project the planning necessary for your life goals. Your wood element gives you growth, stability, creativity, and flexibility to move ahead with your life. The wood element is also a catalyst for your healing. The Liver & Gall Bladder meridians are of the Wood element. Wood is kind when in balance, and angry when not in balance.

- **Fire:** The Fire element is reflected in the energy of summer, and it helps you to mature by energetically embracing your life in a joyful and passionate way. It facilitates your connectedness from the heart in all kinds of relationships. The Heart, Small Intestine, Pericardium and Sanjiao (AKA triple burner)meridians are of the Fire element. Fire is joyful when in balance, and raging when out of balance.

- **Earth:** The Earth element is reflected in the energy of late summer. It is the seat of your intention. This energy enables you to nurture, accept, and support others for the sake of service. It helps you to feel the pain and suffering of others with compassion and thoughtfulness. It assists you in your stability and grounding, so that you can support yourself and others through right action. The Spleen & Stomach meridians are of the Earth element. Earth is satisfied when in balance, and worried when out of balance.Earth element brings stability, strength, comfort and grounding. The person who has balanced their earth element can feel a deep connection with the earth and feel more rooted or grounded. These people are able to be calm and have better thoughts and also can balance their lives. This helps to make sure the energy flows and it removes all the blockages created during the different phases of life. The blockages are created mainly due to greediness, laziness, attention seeking attitude, narrow-minded thoughts and overly materialistic gain thoughts.

- **Metal:** The Metal element is reflected in the energy of autumn. It helps you to let go of attachments on all levels of your being. The metal element helps you to separate the pure from the impure in your world, and to determine your standards. The metal element also connects you to spirit, enables you to "believe", and find meaning and purpose in your life. The emotion of Metal is Grief. The Lung & Large Intestine meridians are of the Metal element. Metal is courageous when in balance, and depressed when out of balance.

Crystals for Reiki

Crystals have been used for centuries as tools for healing and increasing levels of awareness with each stone being specially selected for specific frequencies and properties. Although combining Reiki with the use of crystals is relatively new, this branch of Reiki has the potential to not only transform your current Reiki practice, but our world as well.

Crystal Reiki utilizes the frequencies that reside within the earth and amplifies them through the power of Reiki energy. By infusing these powerful vibrations with the consciousness of Reiki energy, the shifts can be targeted and profound.

The earth vibrates at a specific frequency known as the Schumann resonance. Traditionally this resonance is thought to hover around 7.8 Hz though it varies from region to region. Since 1980's however this frequency has been thought to be rising. This is interesting because science is beginning to understand that we are impacted deeply by the earth's resonance and as it increases, the dissonance between our own frequency and that of the earth is felt deeply on all levels.

These frequencies are thought to impact our autonomic nervous system, brain and cardiovascular system.In your life and the world around you, you may be noticing that things are getting more polarized.

People are gravitating towards the ends of the spectrum with regard to emotions and consciousness. As the frequency of our planet increases, we are given a choice to either raise our own awareness and frequency so that we will feel resonance with earth or to resist it and feel the effects of physical imbalance as well as mental/emotional chaos.

These shifts in the earth's geomagnetic activity are correlated with hospital admissions, death from heart attacks and strokes, as well as many other physical imbalances such as depression, fatigue, mental confusion, and even the number of traffic accidents that occur.

Our body's ability to maintain balance is greatly impacted by the shifts in frequency of the earth. Studies have even connected major political and social events to the earth's energetic activity such as solar flares.

In one study, 80% of the most significant events occurred when solar activity was at its peak. On the flip side, it is thought that just as the frequencies of the earth impact us, our collective frequencies also have a dramatic effect on our planet. There have been studies that show when a group of individuals unite in a state of awareness, the randomness in their environment is reduced.

A study that examined the ability of an individual to affect the DNA was conducted by cellular biologist Glen Rein. The individual's studied were trained to elicit specific emotions such as love and appreciation and then hold a test tube of DNA.

When tested, there was no significant change in the test tube samples. Rein then had a second group of trained individuals create not only the positive emotions, but also hold an intention which in this study was to either wind or unwind the strands of DNA in the sample they were holding. In this group there were significant changes in the DNA with some samples being wound or unwound as much as 25%. The third group of participants were asked to hold only the intention without a positive emotional state and the samples with this group experienced no change.

In this study, the combination of the intention of the practitioner with their own state of presence elicited significant change. Just as thought needs the catalyst of presence to be effective, crystals need the energetic infusion of universal life force to transmit their balancing properties.

The combination of Reiki and the crystals you use will create a unique electromagnetic signature that will send a specific signal out into the field and draw in the information needed to fulfill the set intentions. Crystal Reiki has the potential to connect you with the rising consciousness around you and help you align with it and use it to help yourself and others. As we connect and in a state of presence use Reiki energy to amplify the energy of the crystals we work with, that energy can in turn positively impact the earth so that a symbiotic relationship can be created.

One study demonstrated that even a group of 2,500 individuals taking time to be present through meditation elicited a 25% reduction in crime rates in a population of one and a half million.

In your Crystal Reiki sessions you will not only be in a state of heightened awareness, but you will be harnessing the universal life force energy and using crystals to focus and refine that frequency. As Aristotle noted, the whole is greater than the sum of its parts. Together, within the specific energy field of our work, miracles can occur with the individuals we work with and with our world.

How Crystals for Reiki works

In a Crystal Reiki session, you will use specifically selected crystals and place them in a specific layout around and on the recipient and then allow Reiki energy to flow through you into the crystals and then the recipient. Just as sunlight shining through a crystal prism creates facets of light, Reiki energy passing through the crystals will create a specific energetic resonance within the recipient that their body will then use to address specific imbalances. The presence of Reiki energy amplifies the energy of the crystals and helps the bodymind of the recipient focus on specific areas of the body, conditions or levels of awareness that are ready to heal. In a Crystal Reiki session, Reiki energy is coming from above through the crown chakra while the crystals used in the session bring in a grounding energy from the earth. Together these energies work seamlessly. Crystals are solid symmetrical structures with regularly ordered atoms and molecules that are packed in repeating patterns which extend in all three dimensions of space. The shape and atomic structure of a crystal define it. The defects within a crystal can also define its healing properties and rather than being seen as irregularities, can be intuitively used with powerful effects. Although crystals are considered a part of the mineral kingdom, minerals are less transparent than crystals and darker in color with a consistent chemical structure. Minerals are thought to strengthen the physical aspects of the body such as bones, tissue etc. Both minerals and crystals can be used to help balance the recipient in a Crystal Reiki session. Similarities can be found in the structures of a crystal and our own DNA with dodecahedrons and icosahedrons found in both.The healing properties of each crystal can be associated with the way in which it was formed. Much of the earth's crystals were formed millions of years ago. Crystals are formed in liquid such as magma or water as well as gas that is pushed up from the earth. As the liquid evaporates, the minerals within that liquid bond. The harder crystals are formed within higher temperatures.The geopathic stress that is present as a crystal is formed also has an impact on its healing properties, with enhanced properties present. You will find that the same type of crystal found in different areas with different geopathic stresses will hold different resonances. Regardless of form, crystals have the ability to absorb, channel, focus and emit energy. The energy of Reiki will infuse the intentions of the practitioner and recipient as well as the energetic properties of the crystal to create a unique high frequency.

Crystals can generate energy through a process known as the Piezoelectric effect. This effect occurs when pressure is applied to the crystal which then generates energy. In the same way, if a voltage is applied to a crystal such as *q*uartz, it will bend or slightly change its shape. We all consist of electromagnetic energy. When holding a crystal, your frequency interacts with the crystal, creating a similar type of Piezoelectric effect. The crystal vibrates and the energy it creates can be transmitted to your own internal energy pathways. One key factor that separates Crystal Reiki from general Crystal Healing is the foundational principles of Reiki.

As Reiki practitioners, we understand that our role is to be the observer that holds space for the healing within the recipient to occur. We do not diagnose or prescribe and allow the recipient's body to be the active participant in their healing.

We are also detached from the outcome. Although we set intentions at the start of a Crystal Reiki session and use our intuition as well as our understanding of crystals to focus the energy of the session, we understand that the session will proceed exactly as the recipient's body needs it to and for the highest good of all concerned.

With no expectations, we also do not use our own personal energy in the session. Crystal Reiki sessions instead are an energizing and healing experience for both the recipient and practitioner because Reiki energy is the amplifier in the session. Continued work with Crystal Reiki helps the practitioner to raise and balance their own awareness which extends to all areas of their life and helps to be a healing force in the lives of everyone they touch.

A Crystal Reiki practitioner uses Reiki energy to create a state of presence that is focused and accesses a higher level of consciousness. This presence holds the space for Reiki energy to activate and amplify the crystal energy for a specific purpose so that the desired outcome can be achieved.

Benefits of Crystal for Reiki

Reiki as a standalone modality is extremely effective even without the use of crystals. It is likely though that you have been drawn to Crystal Reiki because you are ready to add the unique energy it provides to your work. Performing Crystal Reiki sessions can help you to focus on specific conditions that clients are eager to have addressed. Not all of your Reiki sessions have to include crystals and you may find when working with a client initially that you choose to perform traditional Reiki sessions.

As the client's healing progresses, you and they may want to hone in one of the specific issues they are concerned with. Crystal Reiki can provide that focus.
In other cases you may find that a single condition is so pervasive in the client's overall sense of wellbeing that it needs to be addressed first before balancing on a widespread level can occur. In these cases you can begin with Crystal Reiki sessions and then use traditional sessions as you feel called to.

Clients who are not in tune with their energy or the frequencies around them may have a difficult time perceiving energy in a traditional Reiki session. Crystals are tangible forms of energy. Although they are beautiful objects that we can hold, they also hold powerful energetic vibrations that can be sensed.

Using crystals can help clients tune into the energetic level which in turn can reassure them that shifts are happening. This reassurance is what helps them to make the conscious choice to return for more sessions and healing. Although in your traditional Reiki sessions you are using your intuition to guide you as you move from position to position and receive information from the recipient's bodymind, in Crystal Reiki your playground has more for you to explore.

You will use your intuition to help you choose the crystals as well as the special layout they will be placed in. During the session you can tune into each crystal for information it may have as well as the combined energies of the crystals as Reiki flows through them. In your traditional Reiki sessions, you likely included grounding techniques for yourself and your recipient at the end and/or beginning of your sessions.

Crystals naturally provide that energy so your sessions will be infused with the higher frequency energy of Reiki as well as the centering energy of the earth. You may also find working with crystals in your distance Reiki practice very helpful. In place of performing a traditional Reiki distance session, you can create a crystal grid connected to the recipient and their needs and allow it to draw in Reiki energy each day.With the foundation of Traditional Reiki with you, you can use Crystal Reiki to take your practice to exciting and wondrous new levels.

The 3 Pillars of Modern Reiki

The three pillars of modern reiki are a great example of a ritual that enhances the reiki session. It allows the practitioner to connect with their higher self along with the reiki source. This formula is broken up into three parts which are; gassho, reji-ho and chiryo.

Within these three pillars are their own individual attributes. When synchronized together, as with any ritual, we gain a deeper connection to that intent.

Reiki is a Japanese healing technique based on the principle that the practitioner channels energy into the patient by means of touch to activate the natural healing processes of the patient's body. The word reiki is made up of two Japanese words: rei meaning "God's wisdom" or "the higher power" and ki which means "life force energy." Reiki restores physical and emotional well-being in a manner that is relaxing and nonevasive to the client.

THE FIRST PILLAR: GASSHO

The first pillar of Reiki, gassho, is more than a meditative practice. It also serves as a form of spiritual hygiene, a ritual to create intention and focus, an invitation to mindfulness, a call to set aside ego, and the primary method to invite and ignite Reiki healing energy within a session.

While gassho is primarily taught in modern forms of Reiki as a meditative practice that entails holding one's hands in prayer position and focusing on where the middle fingertips meet, it is far more involved and deeper than these simple instructions indicate.

During gassho, while the fingertips serve as a physical focal point to help the Reiki practitioner remain mindful and in the moment, a skilled practitioner combines the mindfulness of gassho with breath work and intention.

- **As spiritual hygiene:** As spiritual hygiene, Reiki practitioners should engage in gassho for 5 to 10 minutes before every session in order to purify not only the energy of the space in which the sacred sharing of the Reiki energy will occur, but also to enter into a state of mindfulness where he or she is open to Reiki energy and positive guidance. This is especially important for practitioners who live "normal" lives between sessions (and don't we all?) where the needs of the world often intrude on upon our ideal spiritual state of being.

Before every session, perform any energy work in your healing space you normally do as part of your pre-game ritual, whether that involves burning herbs, drawing symbols in the space, or any other space clearing ritual. Next, sit comfortably in the space in gassho.

Concentrate on your breathing and the space where your middle fingertips meet. Feel Reiki forming in the air around you and breathe it in, allowing it to flow in through your nose and lungs and throughout your entire body.

Exhale tension or anything from your day that does serve you nor not belong in your session. Do this for as long as it takes. Some days, it may only take five minutes, but on those other days where the world has intruded, it may take longer. Do this until you are calm, peaceful, centered, and out of your ego.

Only then should you invite your healing partner into your healing space.

- **To Set Intention, Invite and Ignite Reiki Energy:** Once you have invited your healing partner into the appropriately prepared space, consulted with them as needed, and they are resting comfortably on your treatment table, stand at your partner's head or feet and enter into gassho again. This time, do so focusing on any intention for the session you and your healing partner have agreed upon along with the intention to serve the highest and greatest good. Once again, feel the Reiki gather around you. Breathe it in, and invite it to flow through you and into your hands. When you feel your hands ignite, you can begin your session.

- **To Return to Mindfulness or Seek Guidance:** Throughout your session, you can return to gassho any time you feel the need. Gassho is your safe space where you can return to mindfulness, refocus or reset intention, or receive guidance about where to place your hands on your healing partner. It is the form within the freedom of an intuitive Reiki session. If you feel your mind start to drift or notice your energy shift, return to gassho. If you feel unsure about what to do next, return to gassho. Walk to your partner's head or feet again and stand in gassho until you feel refocused. If you need, ask for guidance and then pay attention. A thought may come into your head, a part of your healing partner's body may "light up" in your gaze, or you may just feel drawn to a certain area. Go with this flow. Return to gassho whenever you need to recenter, wish to return to mindfulness if the outside world starts to intrude on your session, or feel unsure of what to do next.

- **To Give Thanks and Return to Yourself:** You can also return to gassho at the close of a session. When you feel ready, move to your healing partner's feet and stand in gassho. Give thanks to Reiki and to your partner for allowing you to channel the energy to serve the highest and greatest good. Then, invite your energy to return to you and see the energetic connection between you and your partner releasing. When you feel ready, run your hands under cool water or touch the ground to ground yourself.

THE SECOND PILLAR: REIJI-HO

Gassho is interwoven throughout the other two pillars of Reiki. Reiji-ho, the second pillar, is all about asking for guidance. While First Degree Reiki practitioners learn the Reiki hand positions, as they progress they may begin to feel comfortable enough to work intuitively. I encourage students entering Second Degree Reiki to begin working intuitively as often as possible during Reiki sessions knowing if they need to, they can always return to the hand positions.

In reiji-ho, you invite guidance in. It begins in gassho, with your hands held in prayer position asking to have your hands and energy guided to serve the highest and greatest good of your healing partner. And then, you wait and you use all of your senses to listen. Listen to how your body feels, what your mind thinks, what your eyes see, and how your healing partner responds. As you wait for guidance, observe with all of your senses and allow your mind to empty so it becomes a vessel into which guidance can flow easily.

You will learn over time how your Divine Guidance signals you. You may spot a twitch. You may feel something in your own body. You may hear instructions in your mind. You may feel as if you are magnetically drawn to somewhere on your healing partner's body. There is no wrong way to receive information.

Reiji-ho takes trust in yourself, your healing partner, your Divine Guidance system, Reiki, and the universe. It also requires mindfulness. It requires you to allow yourself to be energetically open in order to become a vessel the universe uses to serve the highest and greatest good. When you receive a signal, trust it, act on it, and know the Reiki energy will flow exactly where and as it is needed for the highest and greatest good.

When you feel yourself slipping out of that space as a vessel and a channel and back into your own personal stuff, return to gassho and re-set yourself.

THIRD PILLAR: CHIRYO

The third pillar of Reiki, chiryo, is all about action. Chiryo means "treatment," and it is an essential part of every Reiki session. New Reiki practitioners focus primarily on chiryo, following the mechanical process of placing hands on the body in set positions and trusting the Reiki will flow where it's needed.

However, as a practitioner becomes more deeply involved in the true practice of Reiki, chiryo is something that flows and changes depending on intuitive information the Reiki practitioner receives and the needs of his or her healing partner.

A practitioner truly engaged in chiryo moves beyond the basic hand positions and sometimes even moves beyond use of the hands. He or she may be intuitively guided to gaze, tap, stroke, blow, or visualize along with placing hands, palms, or fingertips in the ways they are guided to do so. In this way, a mindful session of Reiki becomes a flowing dance of energy that involves the practitioner, his or her healing partner, and the entire universe.

How to start Practising Reiki

Not everyone who practices Reiki wants to use their training as a means to make a living. However, serving as a healer can be a very satisfying career. As a Reiki practitioner, you can take pride in your work and make a difference in your clients' quality of life.If you are thinking about setting up a Reiki practice, consider the following tips before getting started.

> ➢ **Get Certified:** There are three levels of basic training in Usui Reiki. You only need to be certified in the first level of training to offer Reiki treatments to clients. You will need to be certified in all levels in order to teach classes and give Reiki attunements to students.

> ➢ **Become Comfortable Giving Reiki Treatments:** It is best not to jump in feet first setting up a Reiki practice until you have a clear understanding of your relationship with the

workings of Reiki. Begin experiencing Reiki on a personal level through self-treatments and treating family members and friends. Experiencing all the inner workings of this gentle, complex healing art takes time. Reiki clears away blockages and imbalances gradually. Allow Reiki to help you get your own life in balance before taking on the task of helping others.

➢ **Choose a Work Location:** Reiki sessions are being offered in hospitals, nursing homes, pain management clinics, spas, and home-based businesses. The benefit of working in a hospital, clinic, spa, or elsewhere is that appointment bookings and insurance claim filings are usually taken care of for you. Most health insurances do not reimburse for Reiki treatments, but a few do. Medicare sometimes pays for Reiki treatments if the sessions are prescribed for pain management. Practicing from a home-based office is a dream come true for many practitioners, but this convenience comes with issues to consider. Do you have a room or area within your home, separate from your normal living quarters, that could be dedicated to healing? Does the residential zone you are living in allow home-based businesses? And, there is also the safety issue of inviting strangers into your personal living space to consider.

➢ **Gather Your Equipment and Supplies:** You will want to invest in a sturdy massage table for your practice if the space you'll be practicing in doesn't have one. If you offer to travel in order to make home visits or give treatments in hotel rooms, a portable massage table will be necessary. Here is a checklist of equipment and supplies for your Reiki practice:

- Massage table
- Table accessories (face rest, bolster, carrying case, etc)
- Swivel chair with rollers
- Freshly cleaned linens
- Blankets
- Pillows
- Tissues
- Bottled water

➤ **Advertise Your Reiki Practice:** Word of mouth is a good way to get started working as a Reiki practitioner. Let your friends and relatives know that you're open for business. Have business cards printed up and distribute them freely at local bulletin boards at libraries, community colleges, natural food markets, etc. Offer introductory workshops and Reiki shares to educate your community about Reiki.

In the modern era, word of mouth also means having a presence on social media. Setting up a Facebook page for your practice is free and only takes a few minutes. Ideally, you'll have your own website that lists your location and contact information, but if that's out of reach, a Facebook page is a good start to draw in new clients. Facebook also has tools that allow small businesses to reach a targeted audience (costs will vary).

➤ **Set Your Reiki Fees:** Research what other Reiki practitioners are charging in your area for their services. You will want to be competitive, but don't undercut yourself. Do a cost-benefit analysis and know how much you need to earn—whether it's per hour, per patient or per treatment—to cover your expenses and have some money left over. If you arrange to treat clients outside of your home, chances are you will either pay a fixed rate for a rental space or share a percentage of your session fees with your host business. Keep good records of the money you are earning. Working as an independent contractor involves being informed of your income tax and self-employment obligations.

➢ **Offer Free Reiki Evenings:** A free Reiki evening can create lots of interest. Plan one night a month to talk about Reiki and give sample treatments. If you have Reiki friends, ask them to come and help give treatments. This is a great way to help others and let them know about Reiki and your practice. Make up flyers for your free Reiki evening and put them up in appropriate places. If the Reiki practitioners can meet an hour or so before the meeting to give treatments to each other it will really improve the quality of what the non-Reiki people receive. Also, if you have taken

Reiki III/master training, you could give a refresher attunement or healing attunement to each of the practitioners to boost their energy. This is a great way for the practitioners to practice their Reiki and for you to practice giving attunements. Call everyone you know who would be interested and let them know.If your area has psychic or wholistic fairs, get a booth. Take a Reiki table and ask 5 or more of your Reiki friends to help. Offer 10 or 15 minute treatments with 5 or more Reiki practitioners giving a treatment to one person at a time. Charge $10.00 or so per treatment. This can be a powerful healing experience and a good demonstration of Reiki. Have a table with your flyers and business cards on it and be sure to get each persons name, address, and phone number for your mailing list. Another way is to use chairs and have one or two practitioners give 10 or 15 minutes for each person.

WHO CAN PRACTICE REIKI

Reiki is easily learned and practiced as self-care by anyone who is interested, regardless of the person's age or state of health. Children can learn to practice, as can the elderly and the infirm. No special background or credentials are needed to receive training.

One of the hallmarks of Reiki practice is its simplicity, it can be learned in about ten hours of in-person training, generally offered in group class formats, and doesn't require knowledge of either subtle bioenergy or healthcare. It is a wonderful experience to receive Reiki from someone else, a friend or a professional, there are many reasons to consider learning to practice Reiki on yourself.

The convenience of self-care is valued not only by people with health challenges, but also by others with busy schedules who are seeking more balance in their lives. Additionally, moments of Reiki practice throughout the day can bring centering and relief from pain, anxiety, and stress as often as needed.

People suffering from anxiety or pain who learn Reiki self-care have the additional empowerment of knowing they are never again alone and helpless with their suffering.

Connections To Chakras

Although Reiki and the chakras come from different spiritual and cultural traditions, they have many things in common. Today, many Reiki practitioners use the 7 chakras as an essential part of Reiki healing.

Although some people find this confusing at first, Reiki and the chakra system have more in common than many people realize.

How does Reiki relates to the chakras?

Reiki and the Chakras

Although Reiki and the chakras come from different spiritual and cultural traditions, they have many things in common. Today, many Reiki practitioners use the 7 chakras as an essential part of Reiki healing. Although some people find this confusing at first, Reiki and the chakra system have more in common than many people realize.

What Is Reiki and How Does it Relate to the Chakras?

Reiki is a form of energy healing that originated in Japan. It was discovered by a Buddhist monk named Mikao Usui, who learned to feel and channel the universal life energy that flows through every being. Every person can learn to use this energy for healing by going through a Reiki initiation in which a master awakens the student to Reiki energy.

Since Reiki was first discovered, it has always used the concenpt of energy centers that allow life energy, known as Ki, to move through the body. In the original Japanese tradition, these points are called tandens. Reiki practice originally focused primarily on one energy center, the Seika tanden, which is located in the lower abdomen below the navel. However, there are three tandens. The other two are located in the upper chest and in the center of the forehead.

The chakras, on the other hand, come from Hindu tradition but have also played an important part in Buddhism. The word is Sanskrit for "wheel," although it is often interpreted more as a vortex or whirlpool in energy healing and yogic traditions. The major and minor chakras make up part of the energetic system often referred to as the subtle body along with Kundalini energy that, once awakened, flows through them and activates them. In some traditions, Kundalini awakening must be passed from master to student in a process similar to the Reiki initiation. The primary focus in energy healing is on the seven major chakras, which run up the center of the torso and head and are the main focal points for the meridians, or energy lines, that run through the body.

The minor chakras are smaller focal points where meridians cross.The tandens and the chakra system are simply different interpretations of the same thing. Essentially, they are points that regulate energy flow. If they are blocked or unhealthy, energy cannot flow freely and illness and discomfort result.

Many Reiki healers use the chakra system instead of the tandens. The chakras provide a more detailed energetic map of the body, allowing the healer to focus his or her energy where it is most needed. Although the concept of meridians and energy flow are the same in both systems, the fact that there are seven major chakras can make it easier to provide specific Reiki treatment for physical ailments.

Chakra healing can also help focus emotional and spiritual treatment. The seven chakras each align closely with aspects of mental wellbeing. A Reiki practitioner who has studied the chakra system can use emotional symptoms to help determine where a blockage might have occurred and focus energy on that.Using the chakra system can also help someone who is not a Reiki practitioner take a more active role in their own healing. There are many ways to help balance and open the chakras, including:

- Meditation
- Yoga
- Wearing or using chakra healing stones
- Eating certain foods or spices associated with the chakra
- Aromatherapy

Each chakra has different elements, colors, foods, and asanas associated with it. By incorporating those elements and practices into daily life in conjuction with Reiki treatment, a person can help speed his or her healing process.In addition, many people find the chakra system more intuitive than the tandens. The colors and symbols associated with it can help with visualizing energy flow and give healers something to help sharpen their focus as they work.

How to do Reiki on Yourself and Others

Self Healing or Treatments are very important when it comes to learning Reiki, at any level .In level 1, you are attuned to receive Reiki, and you are thought the fundamental or basics of how to use it for you own healing and that of your friends and Family.

It is important that you first use it on yourself, for your own self healing and development . Reiki is pure love , it is an act of love to give yourself a Reiki treatment everyday. How many of us, could to do with this in our lives, by giving ourselves 15-30 minutes healing everyday, we give ourselves priority .

By treating on a daily or regular routine, you are keeping the flow of energy flowing through body, which is helping your own healing, by aiding your natural immune system, releasing blocks, this also helps you to understand your own body and helps to improve your intuition, Physically , Energetically , Emotionally and Spiritually you will feel a lot better.

- **Taking Responsibility:** When we give ourselves Self Healing Treatments, we are also taking responsibility for our own healing on every level, even though Reiki can not cure everything, it helps to promote and prioritize our own healing and needs, it does this by teaching us to love our selves unconditionally, it helps us to make changes in our lives, that benefit our health and Well-being . You have often heard the saying " in order to make way for the new, some or all of the old behaviour patterns have to be removed" , and this is what it does , he helps you to realise what's not serving you, and helps you to release it. It trains you , to start looking after yourself, by respecting every aspect of your health and Well-being, helping you to be Happier, Healthier, Physically , Emotionally and Spiritually. When we do this, we are in a much better place, to attract what ever we want in our lives, and this includes helping and treating others, and by showing others how to do the same. This is one of the main Reasons why Doctor Usui started training other people to do Reiki, he found that in early days, the same people kept coming back to him for the same treatments, and they weren't taking responsibly for their own health, so he decided to train some of his clients in Reiki, so they could take responsibility for their health, by using self treatments.

- **Administering Reiki on yourself:** Here for the purposes of First Degree , Level 1 Reiki will show you how to do two Self Treatments, The Heart and Solar Plexus , which some refer to as the Generic Hand Position for Self Treatment, and a Full Self Treatment.

- **The Heart and Solar Plexus:** In this position you place your Left Hand on Your Heart Chakra and Right Hand on your Solar Plexus, you then Ask and Intend for the Reiki to flow to you , for your highest and greatest, and Say Reiki 3 times, Listen to some music, Sit in Peace, Listen to or Say Affirmations for 15 minutes. Its very easy because you can do it at work, on the bus, When you get up in the morning, or just before you go to sleep at night. Its a very Comforting and Reassuring Treatment, and it also connects you to your Hearts Desire.

- **Clearing and shielding:** This is something you can do on a daily basis, especially if you have been around people a lot, or around harsh situations, or Negative people. The First and Easiest Method, is Sit Quietly and Meditate for a Few, minutes , Just to Clear your mind of any internal Chatter, When you have achieved this, take a few deep breaths, and wait, you can feel the Negative or Harsh Energies leaving your with different Sensations, Tingling, or Shivers, or tiny aches and Pains, and your mood gets better and you feel more energised.

Performing reiki on others

You can start healing other people right after being attuned to Reiki degree 1.

As a Reiki 1 channel, you will have to be near the patient you are healing.
After Reiki 2, apart from hands-on healing, you can send anyone Reiki, no matter which part of the world they are.

- **Hands on Healing:** When you are giving hands-on healing to someone, you can either ask them to sit, or lie down. Making them lie down is the most convenient, both for the healer and the patient, as the healer gets comfortable access to all chakras and the patient can relax completely.If the patient communicates with you in advance, ask them to wear comfortable loose-fitting clothes. Once they come for the healing, ask them to remove their spectacles, watch, jewelry, belt, etc. Gold and silver jewelry may be worn. Make sure you and the patient both drink a glass of water. Ask them to lie down comfortably on their back and close their eyes. Start by healing the crown/brow chakra, and then continue to heal all the front chakras.

Once done, balance the energy by spiralling. That is, keep your left hand on their right shoulder, and with your right hand (Index and middle finger extended, thumb touching the ring and little finger) draw anticlockwise spirals starting from the left shoulder, to the tip of the left hand. Next, draw the spirals from the left shoulder to the left foot, then from the right shoulder to the right foot, and then, right shoulder to the tip of right hand.

Ask the patient to turn over the right side and lie on their stomach. Heal the back chakras.
The next step is balancing. Hold your hands above the back brow and back root chakras, about 6 inches above the body. Try to feel the imbalance of energies, and give Reiki till the energy levels feel the same.

Then move your hands slowly to the back throat and back hara chakras. Reiki. Once these chakras are also balanced, move slowly to the back heart and back solar chakras. When these two chakras are balanced, bring both your hands over the back heart chakra and rest it over the body. Keep your left hand on the patient's left shoulder. With the index and middle finger of your right hand, form a V shape and draw a line from the throat to root chakra.

If the patient is diabetic, then draw a line from the root to the throat chakra. Rest your right hand on his/her back hara chakra. Do this thrice. Gently awaken the patient.

- **Distance Healing:** Distant healing can be done by channels who are attuned to Reiki 2 or above. When you are giving distant healing to someone, it is better to ask them to set some time apart to receive the energy you send them. This increases their energy absorption and will to heal themselves. Ask them to sit with their eyes closed, bare feet touching the floor and without crossing their hands or legs. Let them try to feel the energy coming to them.

There are several ways of sending distant energy. You could use an object as a surrogate, a photograph, an intention slip, imagine them, or send them reiki through your third eye. Each of these points is covered in detail.

Distance Healing Techniques

- **Using a Photograph**: You could ask the patient for a photograph and send reiki energy to the same. Draw the symbols at the back of the photograph and if there is enough space, you might even write above it that their problem is solved. Hold the photograph between your palms and imagine the symbols on it while giving Reiki.

- **Using a Surrogate:** You could use a stuffed toy or a similar object as a surrogate. Mentally declare the toy to be the patient and start giving it Reiki. You can give Reiki to the affected part or give full body Reiki to it. You could also declare small objects or your thumb as the patient, and hold it between your palms and give reiki.

- **Imagination:** Keep your palms cupped together and imagine the person either inside your palms or in front of you, receiving the energy you send and bathing in it. Imagine them feeling better, and draw the symbols while giving them reiki.

- **Third Eye:** If the person is visible, you can imagine reiki energy coming through your third eye and going to that person. Imagine a beam of Reiki coming out through your third eye, and draw the symbols on them with that beam. You could use this technique when you are looking at their photograph or simply imagining that they are standing in front of you and receiving reiki through your third eye.

- **Intention Slip:** You could have an intention box, something which can fit into your palm and contain rolled up papers. Take a small chit of paper and write your intention on one side. Take care to use only positive words (avoid using 'no', 'not', 'don't', 'won't', 'can't', etc), avoid any full stops (period .) and don't fold the paper. After the intention, end it with 'It is so, Thank you Reiki, Thy will be done'. On the opposite side of the paper, draw all the symbols. Roll it up and put it in the intention box. The advantage of the intention box is that you can give Reiki to a lot of people/ events at the same time. Whenever you wish, hold the box between your palms, mentally draw the symbols on it and give Reiki. You don't have to think of all the intentions individually.

Reiki Treatments

Reiki treatment that works with energy typically falls under the energy healing umbrella. Each provides similar rebalancing and relaxation benefits. Having said this, there are differences in the theoretical foundations and how practitioners are trained. Energy healing tends to use touch techniques that require healing powers from the therapist themselves.

Therapists will then channel energy into the recipient to bring about healing. Energy healers (sometimes referred to as spiritual healers) may believe they are more vulnerable to other entities, picking up negative energy from the person they are working on.

They therefore need to carry out steps to protect themselves. Reiki healers are believed to be protected by the attunement process.

The calming effect of a Reiki treatment is also beneficial to pregnant women, supporting them on their journey. Children and even animals can benefit from Reiki as it relaxes and soothes.

Promoting a sense of well-being, many find Reiki encourages and supports positive lifestyle choices. Some even say it helps to reduce the need for alcohol and tobacco. When used in conjunction with medical treatment, rebalancing energy can help to manage symptoms of anxiety, fatigue and pain. Reiki can be used for short-term problems or in an ongoing capacity to promote overall health and well-being. Reiki is a natural treatment there are no contraindications, meaning it is generally safe to use for everyone.

You are advised however to discuss your medical history with your Reiki practitioner in case they need to take extra precautions.

Reiki treatments feel wonderful. It's as if there is a warming and healing sensation flowing through the body and the area surrounding the body. As this sensation flows through the body the person can actually feel the stress and illness leave the body.

The key to Reiki is that it treats the entire body, this includes the emotions, the mind and the spiritual portion of the body as well as the physical portion of the body. As the muscles of the body relax, the energy begins to flow freely and the person begins to feel "lifted up" and lighter.It focuses on helping the patient to relax and get in tune with their innermost being. It focuses on letting the world go and bringing in the light of peace and health.

A Reiki treatment instills peacefulness and relaxation into the person's very being. It's soothing, healing and relaxing.

A typical session of Reiki

Before you begin your treatment, your Reiki practitioner will explain to you what the treatment involves. During this consultation, they may ask you why you are seeking Reiki and details of your medical history. Providing as much detail as possible here ensures that they treat you safely and to the best of their ability. After this consultation you will be asked to sit or lie down in a comfortable position.

You do not need to remove your clothing for Reiki treatment. For comfort you may wish to remove constricting layers, shoes and/or glasses. The treatment itself involves the practitioner placing their hands gently on the body, or slightly above the body, in a predetermined sequence. The position of the hands is non-intrusive and should not cause any discomfort.

If you feel uncomfortable at any point, let your therapist know. The amount of time spent in each position will depend on the nature of your concern. The touch should be gentle and light, Reiki is not supposed to manipulate or massage.

Everyone will respond differently to Reiki treatments depending on their individual circumstances. Some people say they feel sensations during their Reiki treatments, while others do not. Some feel heat or tingling during the treatment and some report seeing colours. For some, the experience brings up an emotional response. The most common response however is a feeling of calm, relaxation and well-being.

After the treatment you may feel very relaxed, or you may feel energised. There is no right or wrong way to experience Reiki. Some people say after the treatment they encounter a 'healing reaction', like a headache or flu-like symptoms. If you are concerned about any reaction, speak to your practitioner.

Understanding Auras

For many millennia of human history, it has been a widespread belief that all objects, especially human and animal bodies, have an Aura (or electromagnetic (EM) field), and that this Aura can be visible to the trained eye. Late 19th century metaphysical science expanded on this concept with the theory that all things possess a body of etheric substance, commonly called the Ethereal Body, which is composed of the higher fre*q*uencies of subtle energy and finer pre-matter *q*uantum particles which are intimately bound up with the physical body, as a product of creation of matter by electrofield manifestation through the quantum particles onto the physical plane.

Considering the mechanics of subtle energy fields and energy-matter interactions developed in the late 20th century academic sciences of Bioenergyinformatics and torsion field physics, and given the advanced state of modern scientific instrumentation, it seems both reasonable and logical to conclude that the Aura can be quantified and tangibly studied in an experimental manner. Indeed, since colors of light are defined by frequency, subtle energies and the bioenergy that emanates from all living things can be quantified as electromagnetic field energy that resonates with different frequencies of light.

In fact, much has been learned this century about the light properties of subtle energy fields and Auras from the works of such prominent scientists as the Polish doctor Iodko-Narkovitz, who worked with photo-electricity and electrical field measurement, the Russian inventor Semyon Davidovich Kirlian, who experimented with the qualities and meanings of Auras using photography and electrofield imaging, and the British doctor Walter J. Kilner, who eventually invented a series of goggles and filters through which anyone can see Auras in detail. Many people are also aware.

Currently the list of inventions using subtle energies as treatments and subtle energy detectors is so long that we could not possibly discuss them all.

Many scientists and doctors have been particularly intrigued by metaphysical scientists' claims that the Aura's energy-information can be used to accurately analyze a patient's psychological and emotional states. Current research further suggests that certain levels of bioelectrical Aura fields are characteristic of the physical status of the biological organism. Biological activity such as autonomic responses initiate cellular and electrochemical changes, thereby creating an environment thermodynamically favorable to the conversion of metabolic kinetic energy into electromagnetic energy.

In this process, localized bioenergy "complexes" to form a dynamic field that differentiates according to the neurological information that stimulated it. Since the skin is no barrier for such electromagnetic energy, the bioenergy field can and does radiate outside of the organism to become what we call the Aura.

The Aura is highly characterized and affected by the emotional and physical condition of a person, the biological homeostasis or imbalance of plant life, or the molecular energies inherent in and surrounding an object. This makes the reading of Auras a very useful and powerful tool for the metaphysical and clinical analysis of humans, animals, plants and objects.

The color frequencies of light of which the Aura consists are too high to be perceived by the naked eye in most cases. However, the trained practitioner can learn to perceive these frequencies naturally, by activating the Pineal Body and adjusting their brain waves to the higher frequencies of which the Aura consists.

Most psychics and metaphysical practitioners tend to see the Aura in six basic colors: red, orange, yellow, green, blue, and purple. Although the Aura itself consists of frequencies higher than those in the visible light spectrum, the electromagnetic energies in the Aura have lower, subharmonic frequencies that resonate with the frequencies of each of the colors of the visible light spectrum.

Therefore, although Auras are not visible to the naked eye, the brain may perceive the energies in resonance with certain colors, and thereby construct a quasi-visual (mental) image of seeing those colors. It is precisely in this way that humans sometimes see the Aura, and can analyze its different colors.

Seeing the Aura and interpreting its colors has been the focus of popular metaphysics for centuries, and "What color is my Aura?" is a very popular game in metaphysical and spiritual circles. However, most people "see" colors that do not match the objective frequency color of the actual Aura.

This is because they make a psychologicalassociation between the "feeling" of the Aura energy, and what the color "feels" like intuitively. The associated color is then induced magnetically into the visual center of the brain, so the person "sees" that color while looking at that part of the Aura. As a result of this common psychological phenomenon, the vast majority of literature on Auras and Aura colors are entirely subjective to the psychology of the authors, and the purported meanings of the colors are almost entirely arbitrary.

Structure of the Aura

All interpretation of the objective Aura colors is conditional upon understanding the structure of the Aura itself. Each part and level of the human Aura is related to different aspects of the person's psychology or physical health, and sometimes reveals an interaction of both physical and mental factors. By understanding the structure of the human Aura, we can study the objective meaning of the Aura colors in context.

It is currently unresolved exactly how many "levels" there are to the human Aura. Clinical studies of the human Aura at ITEM, however, indicate that the metaphysical being of a living incarnate entity consists of four basic Aura Bodies.

The highest of the Aura Bodies is the Causal Body, which is traditionally described as our spiritual "higher self" related to our deepest personal identity. Current metaphysical science of the describes the Causal Body as the direct piece of high-frequency universal subtle energy which is given individual consciousness and manifests as an entity which can exist in the physical world of matter. Traditionally called the psyche, or the soul, the Causal Body is the primary subtle energy field that comprises our metaphysical being, and contains our deepest consciousness.

The Causal Body may be detected at about 24 inches above the head and shoulders and beyond.
The next identifiable level is called the Ethereal Body, which is related to the pre-matter quantum particles which are animated and influenced by the Causal Body's electrical life-force energies.

This body also contains imprints of all the temporal energies and *q*ualities that we acquire while incarnate, and which make up our personality. According to ancient theories of reincarnation, these imprinted energies can later be incorporated into the basic Causal Body if they will be for potential successive incarnations.

The Ethereal Body reflects our identity, and consists of the more stable average of our general energies. In general, the Ethereal Body can be detected 18 to 24 inches away from the physical body. Because of its distance from the physical body, this level of the Aura plays an important role in how we interact with other people, because it comes in contact with the ethereal energy bodies of others, and participates in mutual energy-information exchange, both projecting and receiving energy.

The third, and most clearly identifiable, of the four basic Aura Bodies is called the Emotional Body. This is the most useful level for scientific interpretation and analysis, because it is highly characterized by the emotional and psychological condition of the subject. Generally, the Emotional Body can be detected 4 to 18 inches away from the physical body. Because of the wealth of psychological information that can be obtained from this level of the Aura and used to gene-rate a thorough psychopersonal profile, in RFI tech-nology it is regularly referred to as the "Psychological Level."

The Health Level of the Aura, being the fourth and most tangible of the Aura Bodies, is essentially the subtle energy that radiates from the physical body. This most naturally visible part of the Aura is the bioenergy field that emanates from the cellular, neurological, and other biological functions of the physical body.

The Health Level thus reveals the physical condition of the subject, showing disturbances and patterns related to illness or other biological conditions. In general, the Health Level can be detected approximately 0 to 4 inches away from the physical body.

LIVING IN HARMONY WITH

THE WORLD

One of the most essential conditions for people is to feel free and happy and to enjoy life – to be in harmony with one's self and the world. Most people realize the need to cope with their internal conflicts and struggles, to free themselves from negative feelings, to be faithful to themselves, and to live according to their principles – to be at peace with themselves.

Achieving harmony with the world, however, often seems difficult and even unattainable, especially when the circumstances and the people around them are not what they want them to be.It seems as if there is some contradiction in being true to one's self and at the same time being in harmony with the world this individual doesn't like.

So, in this case, people's views, imaginations, and dreams are different from the reality around them. Is it possible to live in agreement with your world, since your desires and aspirations are in conflict with reality? Does it mean that you have to give up on them to be in peace of mind? Or do you have to wait for circumstances to change, to get to the place where you have always dreamed of being and everyone around you friendly and loving to be in harmony with the world around you?

If you set such conditions, you will become too dependent on the outside, and you will never be satisfied. You can only be in harmony here and now, not once when things have become "better", and you do not have to give up your desires and dreams, you do not have to deny the desire to change your lives.

Living in harmony with yourself and with the world are inextricably linked and cannot be separated from one another. There is no way you can be in a spiritual balance if you present yourself against the life you live in. If you hate the people around you, if you cannot forgive those who have hurt you and have caused you pain and anger you will not be able to have a harmonious relationship with others if there are unresolved conflicts and struggles inside you and you are not aware of your own self.

If you want to live in harmony with the world that means you have to be in harmony with yourself. Spiritual peace is achieved when one finds a balance between the external and the inner world.

WHAT YOU NEED TO DO TO LIVE

IN HARMONY WITH THE WORLD

- **Resistance:** Resistance is what mostly pollutes one's inner space and disturbs the mental equilibrium. Resistance creates a constant tension and an internal struggle that tortures individuals and acts as a slow acting poison.Think about it – are you suffering that your life isn't going the way you want it to go, do people around your cause you to be irritated, do you hate your work or the place where you live? What is the reason for all of this? You feel that circumstance and the people around you cause you not to feel well, but actually the real reason is your reaction to them.Because your inner space is the primary reality, and the external is secondary. Imagine, for example, that the colleagues in your work are irritating you, they are behaving badly, they don't appreciate you and are constantly manipulation everyone. Every day, however, you show up to this hateful place, you do nothing different, you curse your fate and inculcate yourself.

The way to deal with the situation, which provokes resistance and negative feelings, is very simple. You have three options: remove yourself from the situation, change it, or accept it totally. If you want to take responsibility for your life, you must choose one of those three options, and you must choose now. Then accept the consequences. No excuses. No negativity. No psychics pollution. Keep your inner space clear." If you cannot leave the situation or change it, then accept it. Realize how pointless it is to be angry at what already exists. Taking the situation does not mean that you will not try to change it in time, but at that moment it is as it is. What's more stupid than hurting yourself, becoming angry and wasting all of your energy in a fight against something that is a fact to turn the enemy into the present.

- **Forgiveness:** when one refuses to forgive, this individual carries a heavy burden within his or her own self. This burden becomes heavier over time. The stench of hatred and negative feelings in this individual grows, con*q*uering the whole body and mind, choking this individual and poising him or her. Run away from the heavy loads of hater. Remove feelings that are torturing you. Remember that forgiveness is for your own sake. By forgiving the people who have hurt you in some way, you are relieved of heavy burdens and cease to perceive and act as a sacrifice. Forgiveness will make you feel free and independent.To forgive does not mean that on the outside you shouldn't take any action. Of course, everyone has to take responsibility for his or her own actions.I am talking about an internal purity that frees you from the painful, self-destructive feelings and makes you live in harmony with the world.

- **Feeling Guilty:** Having a sense of guilt is a very corrosive feeling. From it, one can become sick. It is not by chance that people confess and, having received forgiveness, are released.If you have done something that makes you feel guilty and you cannot find inner peace – do something about it – go to the person who hurt you, speak to them.If you are doing something that makes you feel guilty and you are tortured by these actions, stop doing them.In most cases, to free yourself of guilt, you must forgive yourself. Everybody makes mistakes; no one is perfect. But mistakes are our best teachers. Remember that you have done the best you could at this point. Forgive yourself and move forward.

- **The dichotomy:** The inner divide disturbs harmony and creates stress in life. These are the cases when you are hesitant about what decision to take when you've postponed solving a problem when you break yourself to please everyone, when you have to lie about something,In order to be calm and free, one must have a clear position and act immediately.Don't delay to solve problems. Become involved with them right away. Remember that there are no right and wrong decisions, the only wrong decision is when you do not make a decision, but you postpone.Living in harmony with the world means that you become free.

Myths About Reiki

There are lots of myths prevailing these days related to reiki healing. The idea behind reiki healing is that there is a hidden life force energy flowing inside us that keeps us alive, when this energy gets low in us we easily become sick and when this energy is high we feel happy and relaxed.

MYTH 1: REIKI IS A RELI-

GIOUS ACTIVITY

This perception is totally wrong because Reiki has nothing to do with religion instead it is all about spirituality. The emperor of Japan, Meiji, formed the principles of Reiki. You never find a priest giving sermons on Reiki or church for Reiki. Anyone believing in any religion can take benefit from Reiki treatment.

Reiki absolutely is a spiritual art. The principle teachings of Reiki embrace a life of balance and promotes spiritual growth. But, Reiki is not a religion, nor is it based on any particular religious doctrine. Reiki does not infringe on anyone's beliefs or personal values.

People of many different faiths have discovered the love-energies Reiki offers.

MYTH 2: DR. USUI IS A CHRISTIAN MONK

The founder of the Usui System of Reiki, Dr. Mikao (Mikaomi) Usui, was not a monk, a Christian, or a medical doctor. He was a Japanese Zen Buddhist, a businessman, spiritualist, and scholar. Late in his life, he experienced a profound spiritual enlightenment after a period of fasting and meditation. Afterward, he began the process of developing the healing art of Reiki and opened a teaching clinic in Japan.

MYTH 3: REIKI TREATMENT CAN

HEAL YOU IN JUST ONE SESSION

This is possible but this happens *q*uite rarely. It is said that reiki is not a onetime procedure rather it is a process and in order to see satisfactory results a person should go through 3 to 4 reiki sessions.

MYTH 4: REIKI HEALS AND CURES

If reiki has helped you heal it really does not mean that it has cured you too because healing and curing are two different things. Healing has to do with attacking the root cause of your illness; it is rebalancing of wholeness while curing restores your health by alleviating symptoms of your disease.

MYTH 5: REIKI PRACTITIONER

IS A HEALER

This is not true because Reiki practitioner only acts a medium in the healing procedure. The Reiki practitioner just passes on universal life force to the recipient in order to heal mind, spirit and body of the recipient. Reiki practitioners don't have the powers to heal you they just help you; it is only you who can heal yourself.

MYTH 6: REIKI IS A MASSAGE

THERAPY

Reiki is NOT a massage therapy. Although there are many massage therapists who will incorporate the use of Reiki's healing energies into their massage sessions. Reiki is an energy-based therapy that does not involve manipulating bones or tissues. Reiki practitioners use a light touch with their hands on their clients' bodies or will hover their palms over them. Because it is not a massage, clothing is left on. Although, wearing loose-fitting garments is recommended for your comfort/relaxation.

MYTH 7: GIVING REIKI TO OTHER DEPLETES YOUR

OWN ENERGY

A Reiki practitioner does not give his personal energy over to the client. He serves as a channel, funneling Universal Life Energy through his body to the recipient. Much like the delivery boy delivering a package on your doorstep. The Reiki package is delivered, the delivery boy goes home fully intact. Ki energies are infinite and never run out.

This does not mean that a person giving Reiki may not feel tired after giving a treatment to someone. This sometimes happens and Reiki has been wrongly blamed for it.If a person giving a treatment experiences exhaustion during or after applying Reiki to others, this is likely an indication that something is out-of-balance in his own body or life that needs attention.

Booking a healing session for himself with another practitioner or conducting self-treatments would be warranted.

MYTH 8: HAVING A REIKI ATTU-

NEMENT WILL OPEN UP A DIALOG

WITH YOUR SPIRIT GUIDE

The lure of Reiki attunement, with the promise of a glimpse into the spirit world. Please don't fall for this. This myth may have arisen out of the writings of Stein. In her widely published book she describes how many of her students became aware of who their guides were after months of using Reiki following their level II attunements.

The urban legend that followed was that the attunement alone would make this happen. Some Reiki II classes include a promise to "Meet your Guides." Yes, it could happen and likely has happened for some Reiki initiates, but there is no guarantee.

Conclusion

While some people believe the frequencies associated with the flow of Reiki energy have been superseded by higher frequencies becoming more and more available on the planet. Even so, Reiki continues to remain a very popular and effective form of energy healing. It is safe and well documented and for a lot of people, forms their first introduction to the vast field of Alternative and Complementary healing.

Learning Reiki is a good starting point for experiencing and working with healing energy and it's a wonderful method for deepening awareness of universal healing energies in general. Reiki complements other healing methods and spiritual practices. There are no hard and fast rules about how to approach starting Reiki and Spiritual Healing.

Again, listen to your heart, and you will be guided in choosing the right experiences and the right teacher for you. Once you have learned a healing technique, to work and fun begins. To develop your understanding of, and sensitivity to Reiki, it is a good idea to devote time to regular practice.

Find a supportive teacher and practice group and pursue your continuing study. Make sure that you arrange circumstances so that you can be nurtured in your healing and growth.Keep your eyes on your goals, your mind in your heart and take things one step at a time. Love, light and healing to you on your journey.Practicing Reiki does not appear to routinely produce high-intensity electromagnetic fields from the heart or hands. Alternatively, it is possible that energy healing is stimulated by tuning into an external environmental radiation.

Reiki is an ideal complimentary therapy to go alongside other therapies. They are soothing and relaxing and may prepare the body to accept other medications better. Ideal for anyone suffering from diabetes, AIDS/HIV, high blood pressure, heart conditions and more. Reiki can work hand in hand with modern medicine and enhance the effects of modern medicine. Reiki appears to be generally safe but it should not be used to postpone seeing a healthcare professional!